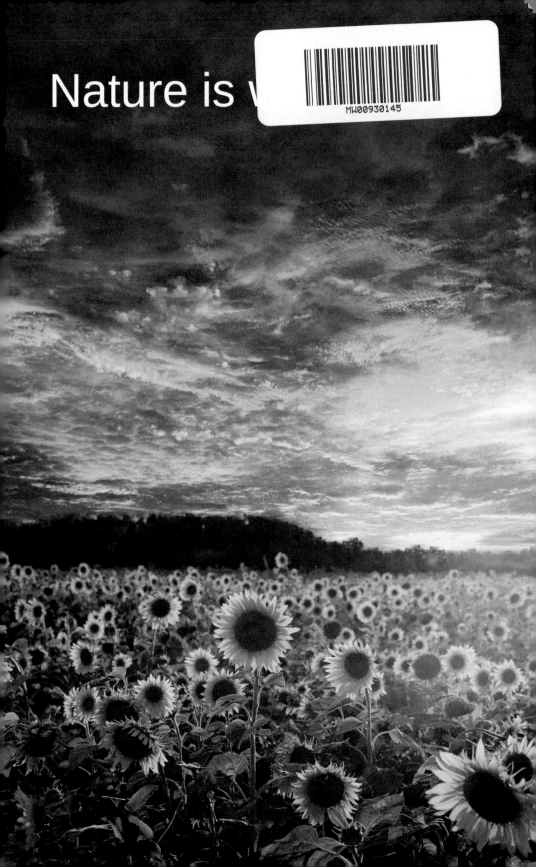

Nature is v

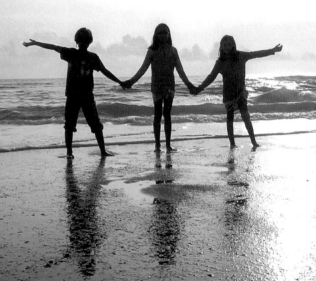

We are all friends.

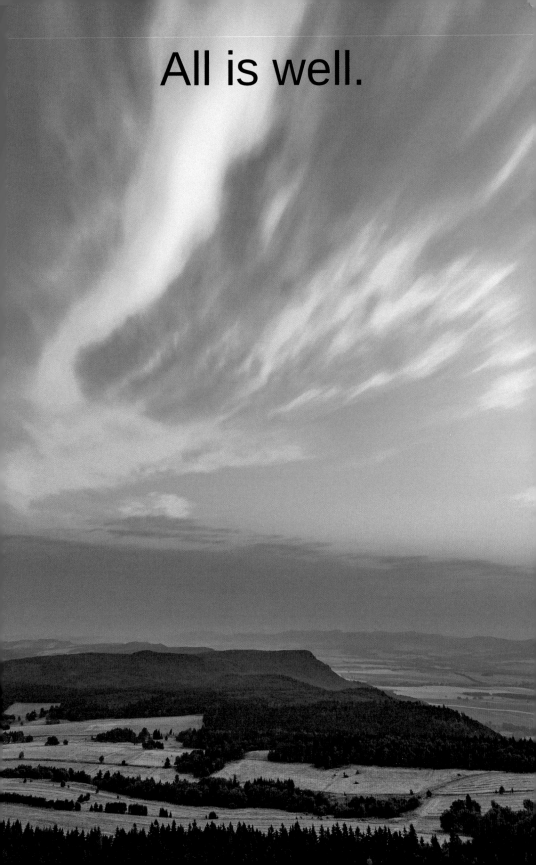

All is well.

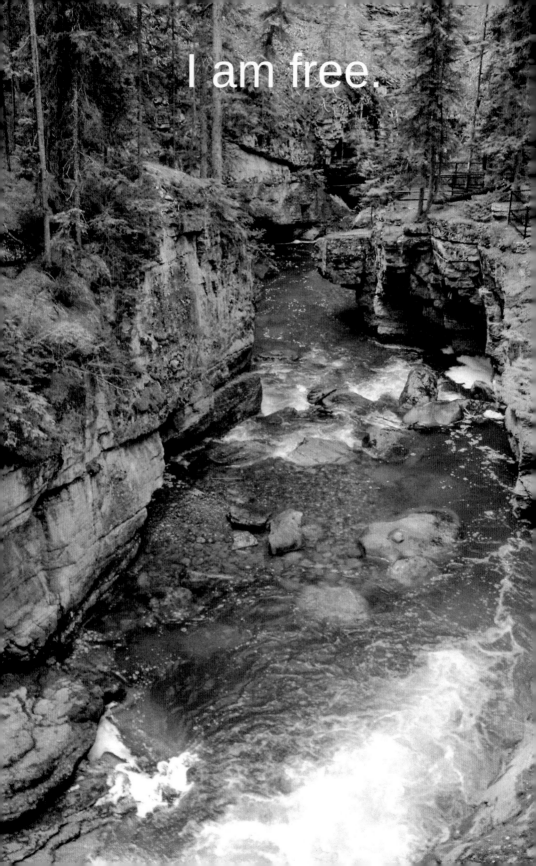

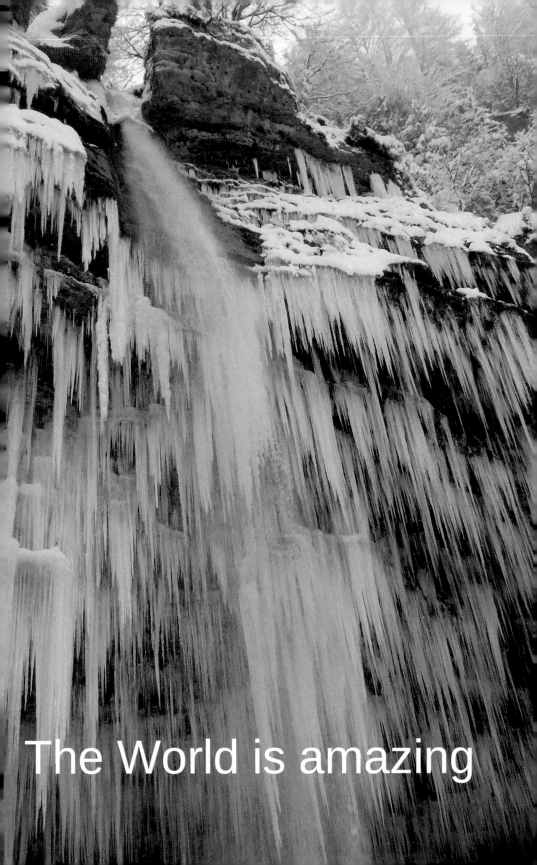

The World is amazing

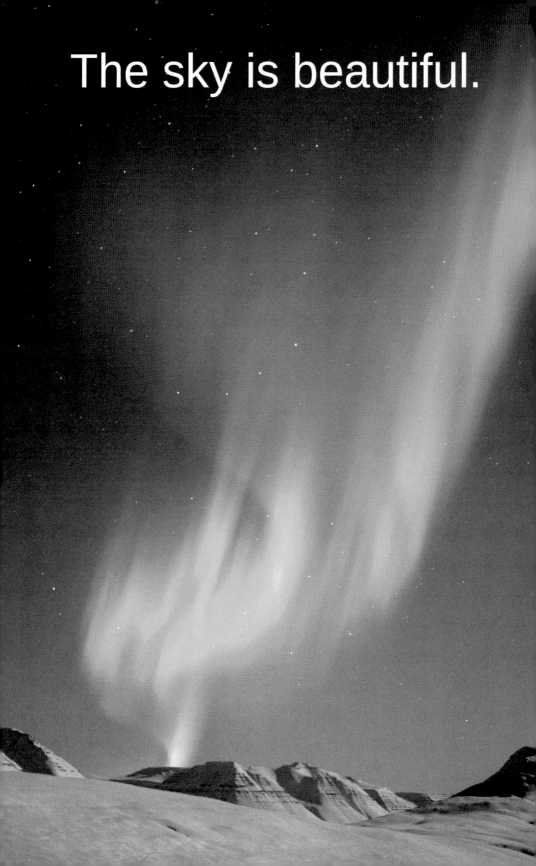

The sky is beautiful.

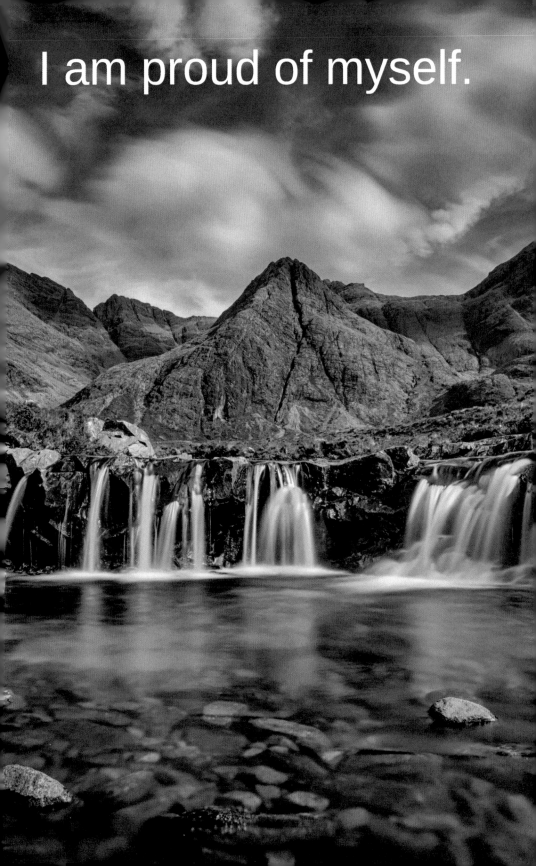

I am proud of myself.

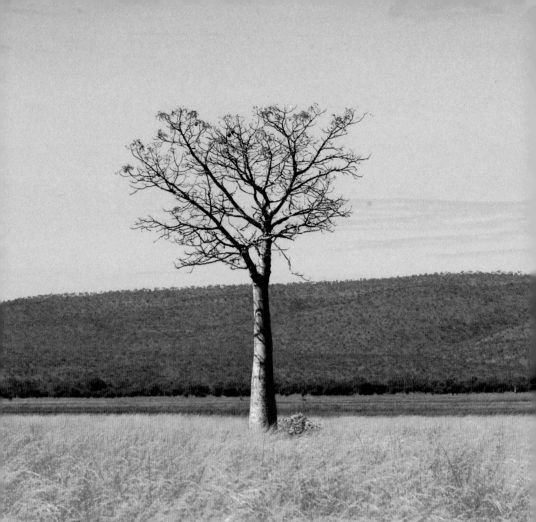

Everything is OK.

Life is peaceful.

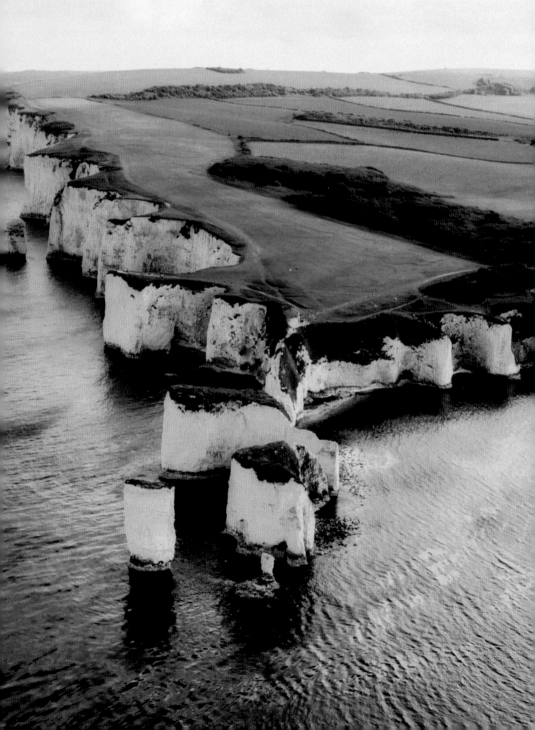

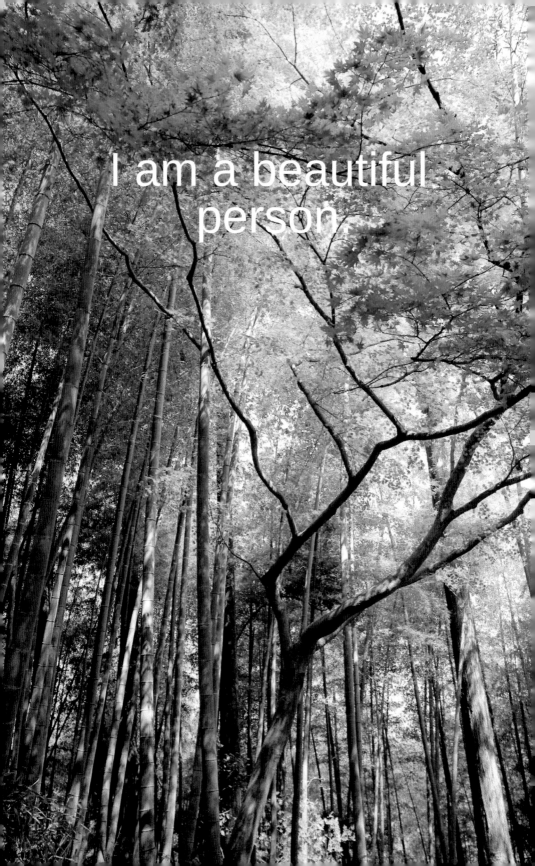

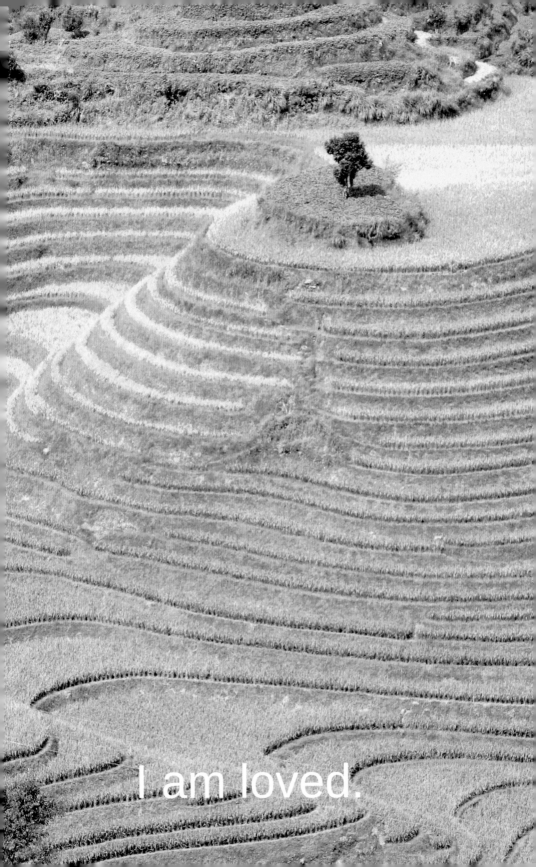

I am loved.

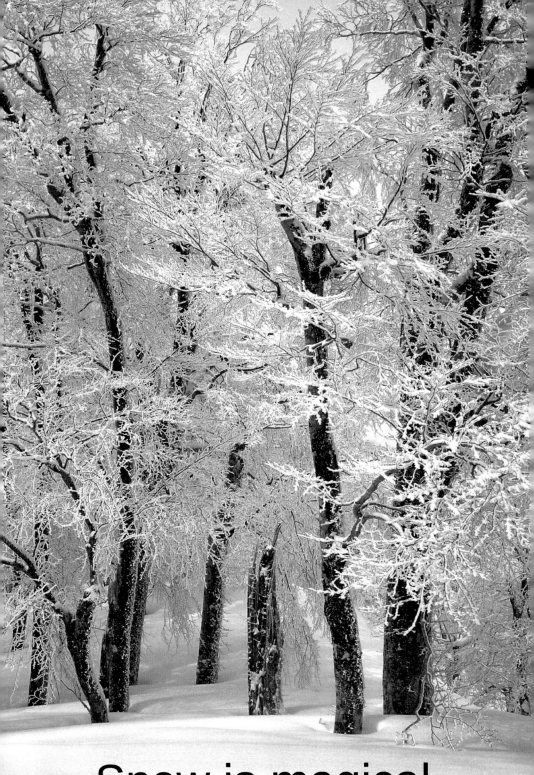

Snow is magical.

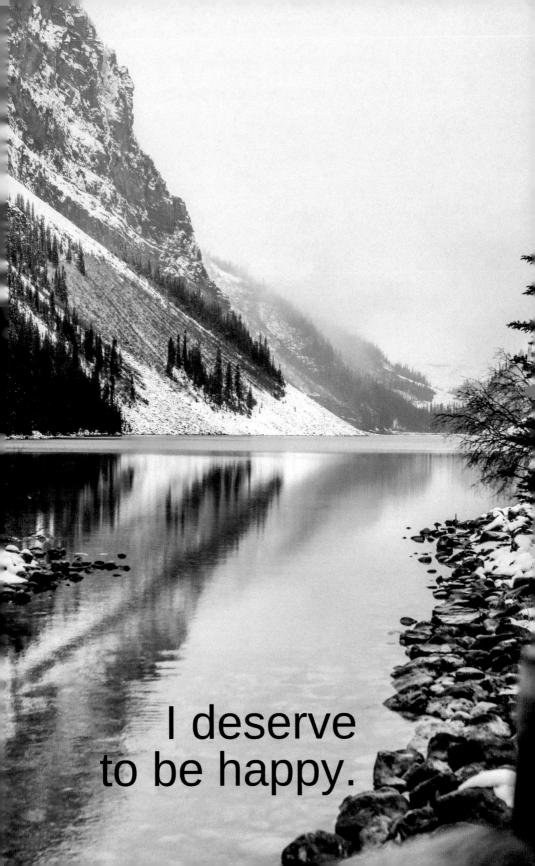

I deserve
to be happy.

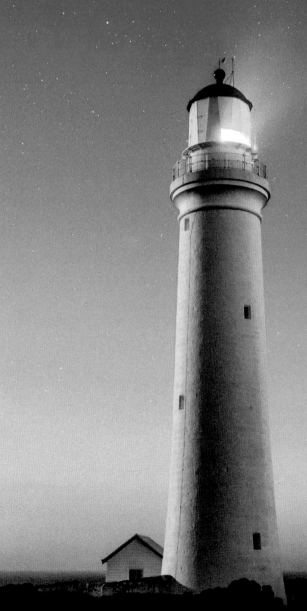

The light keeps us safe.

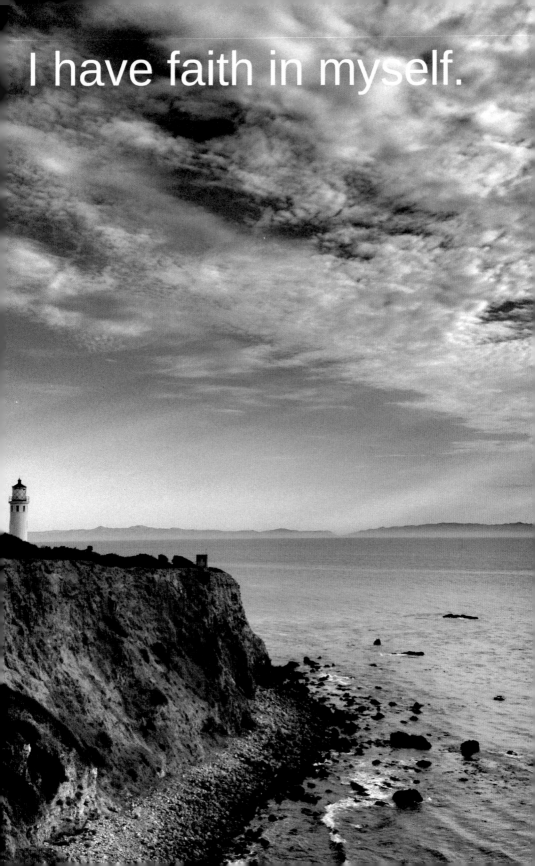

I have faith in myself.

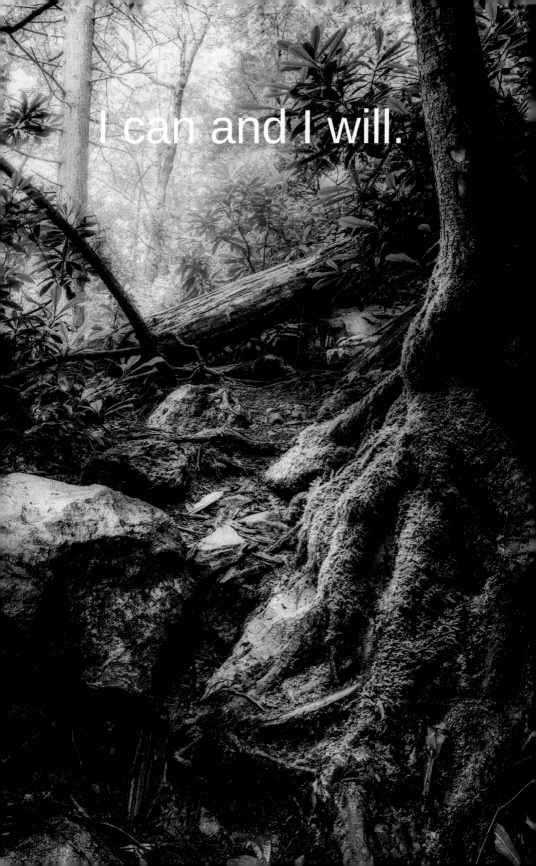

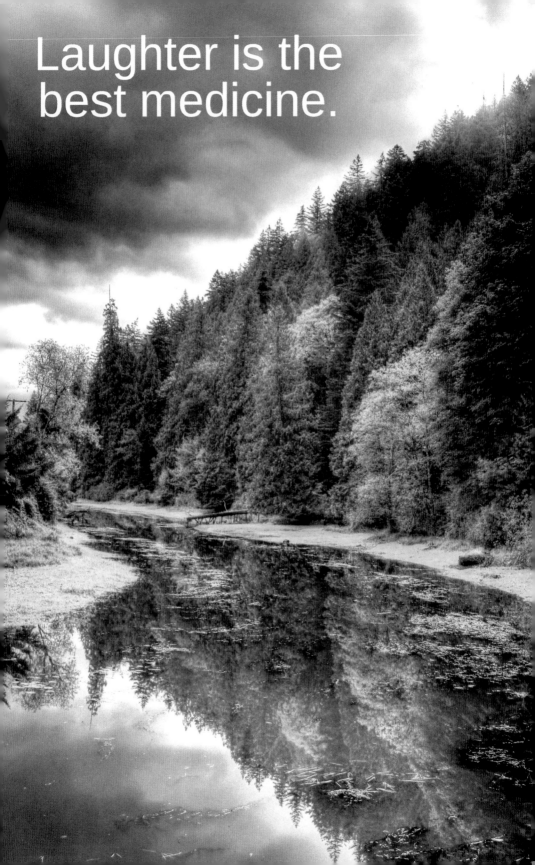

Laughter is the
best medicine.

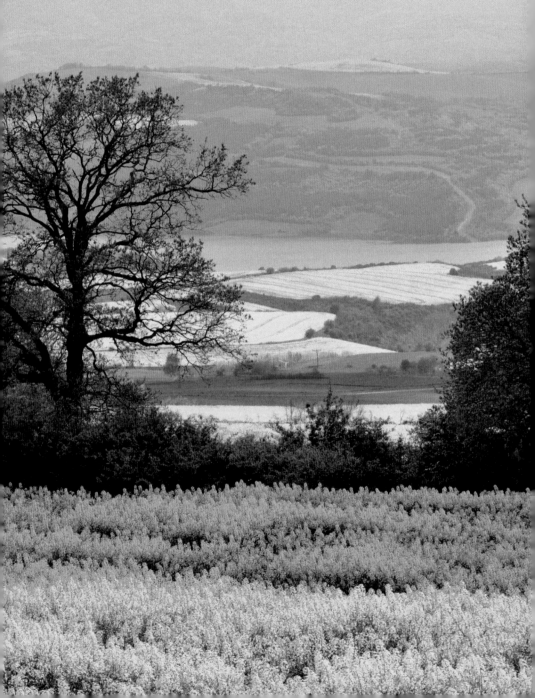

Go with the flow.

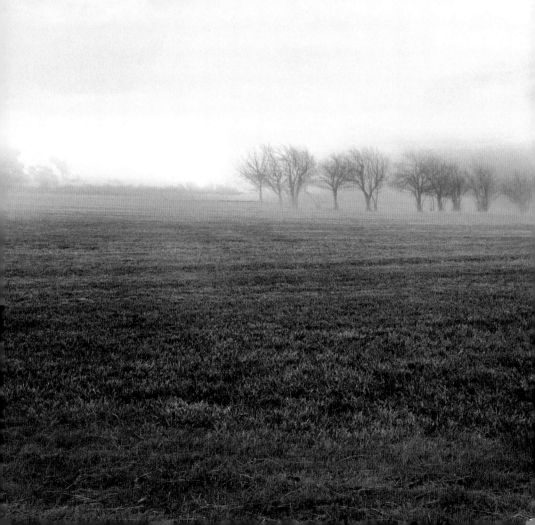

Every day is a
new beginning.

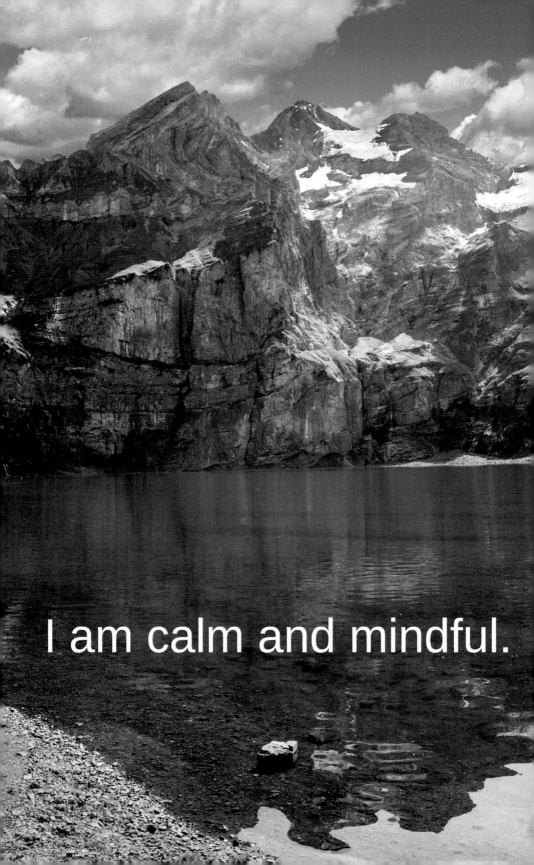

I am calm and mindful.

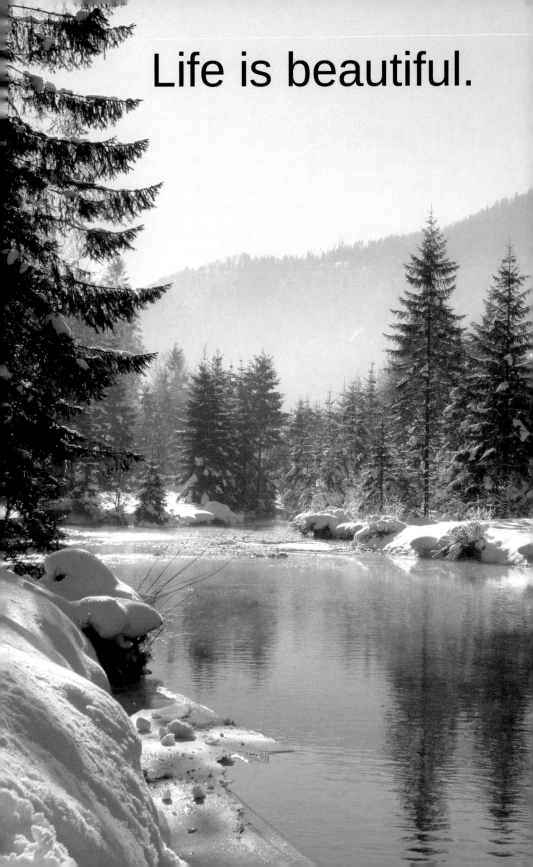

Life is beautiful.

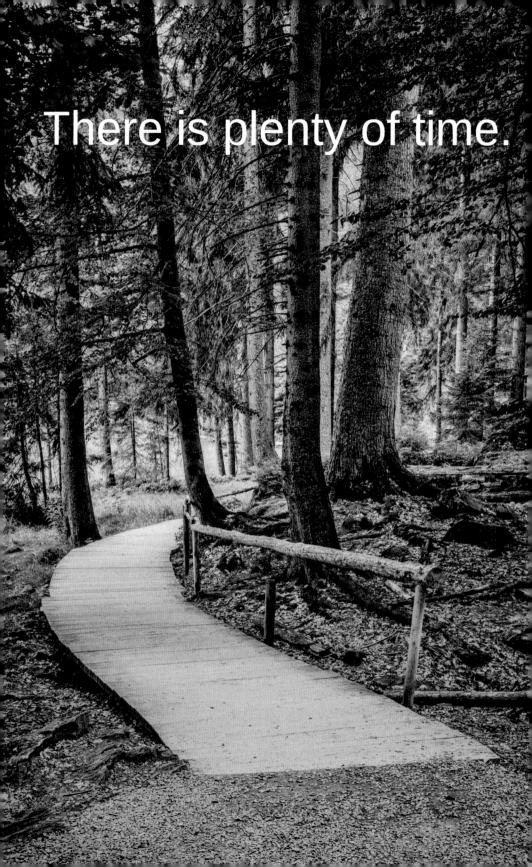

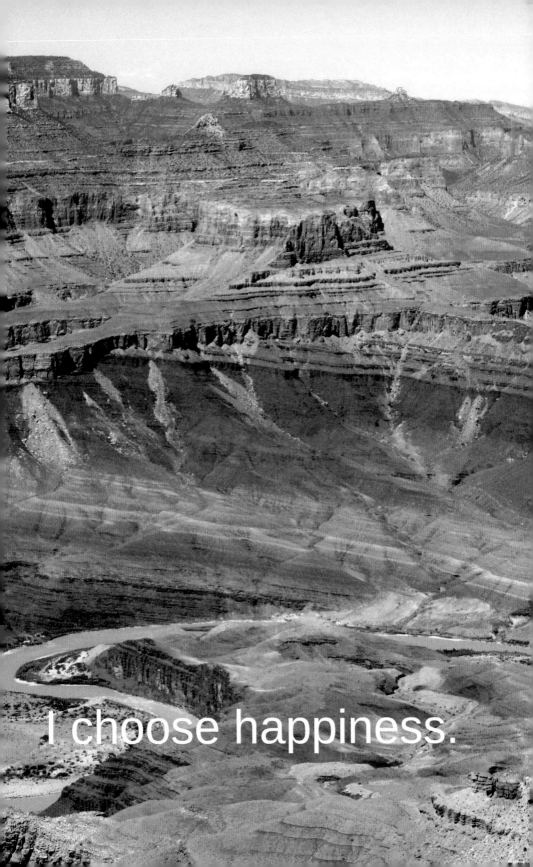

I choose happiness.

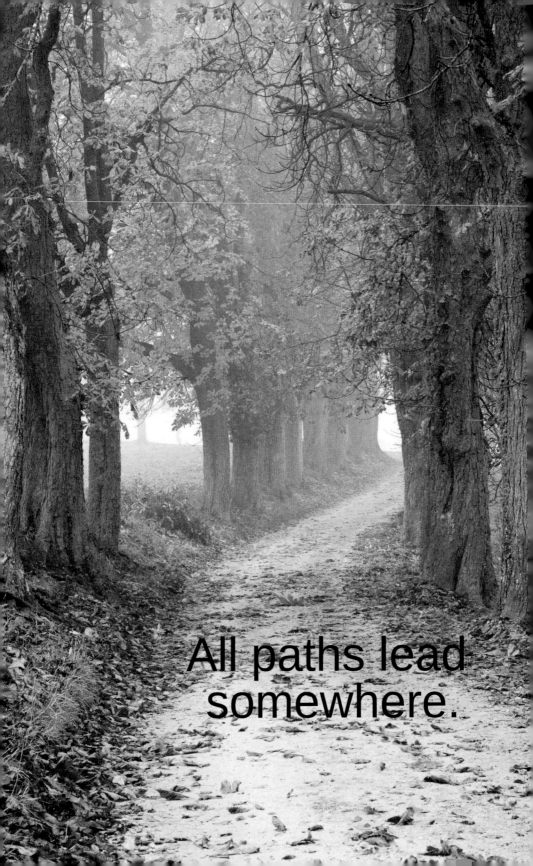

All paths lead somewhere.

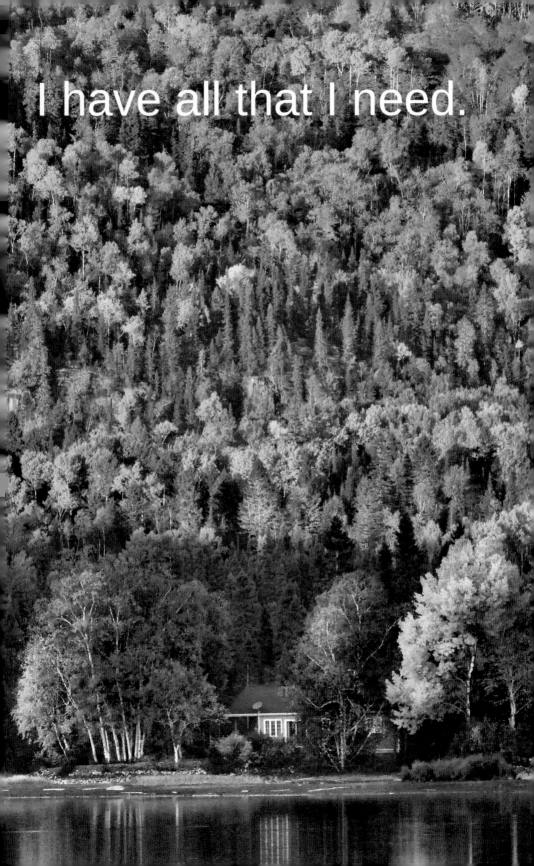

I have all that I need.

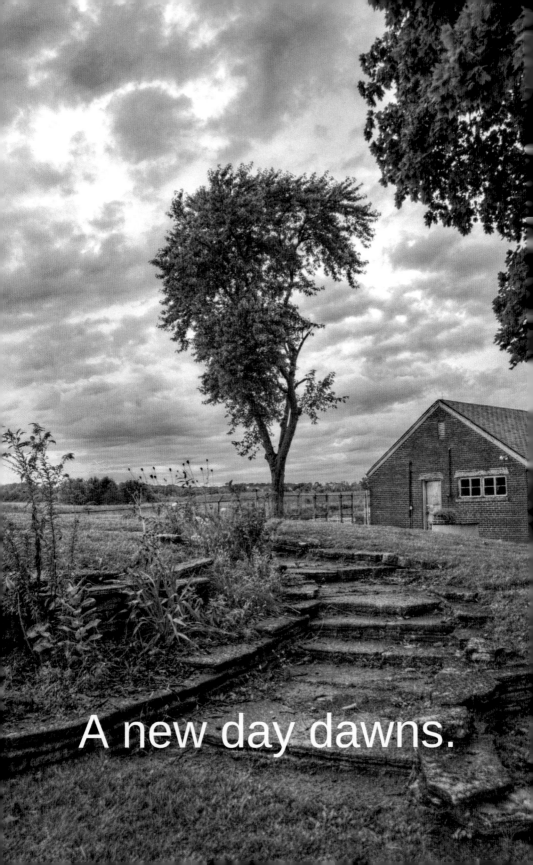

A new day dawns.

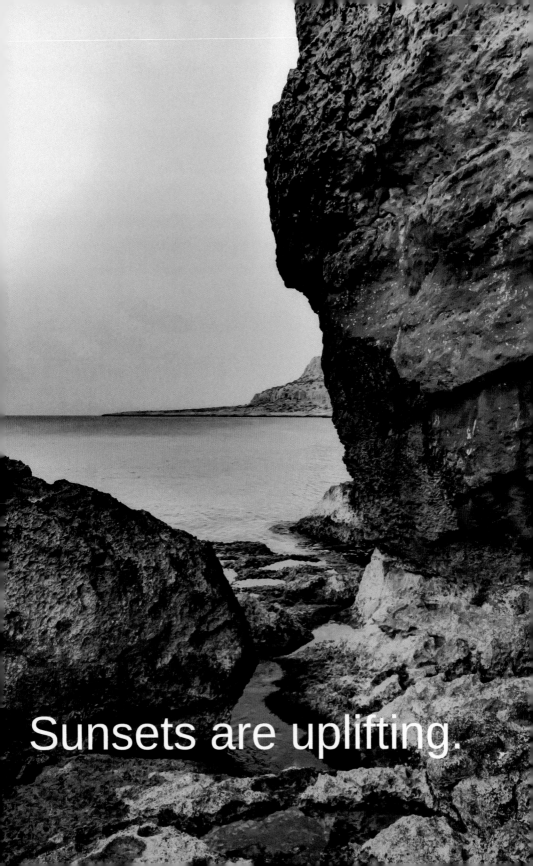

Sunsets are uplifting.

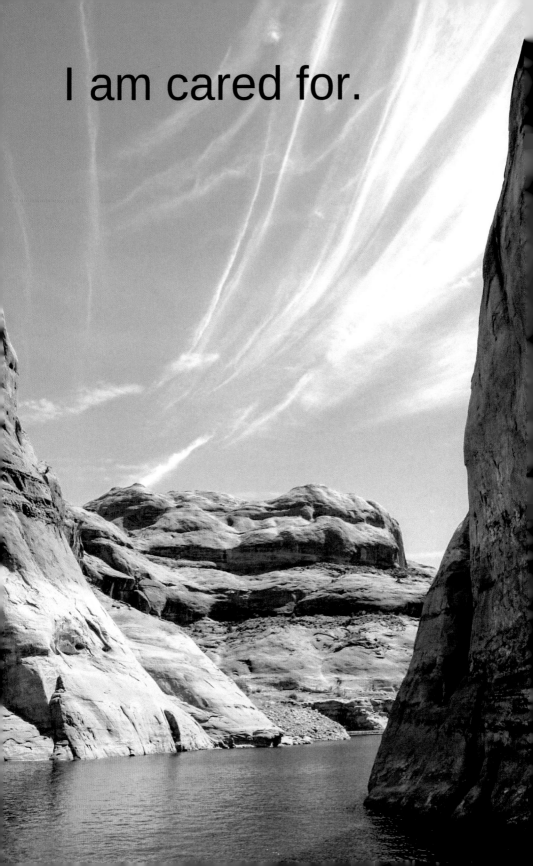

I am cared for.

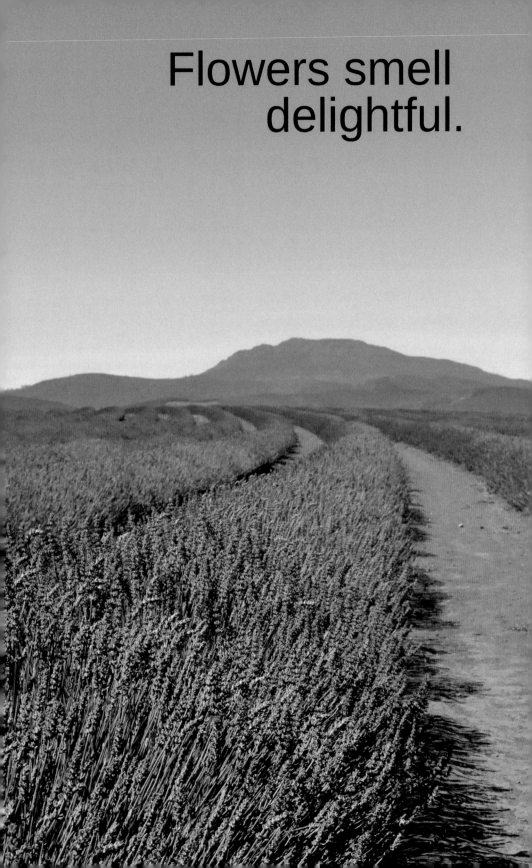

Flowers smell delightful.

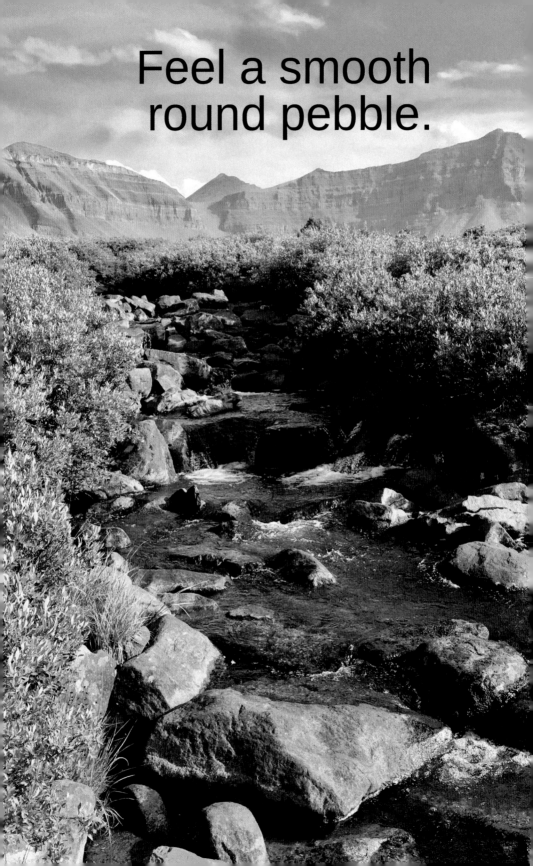

Feel a smooth round pebble.

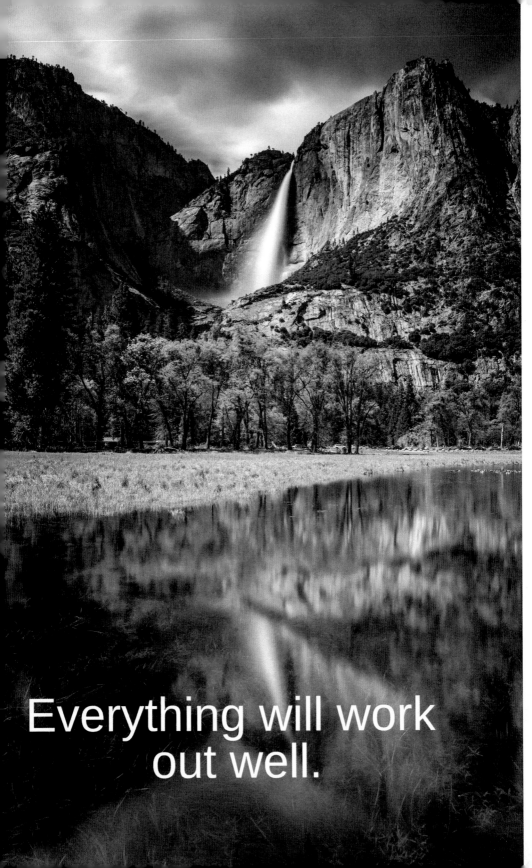

Everything will work out well.

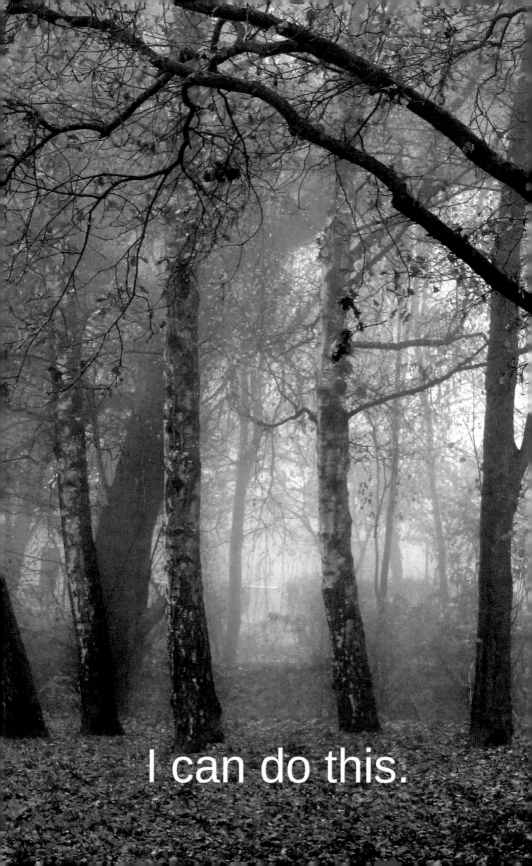

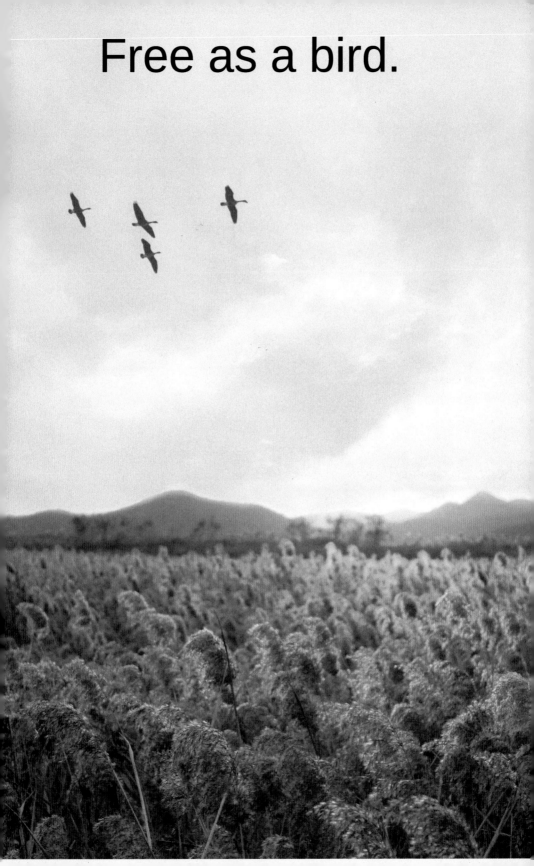

Free as a bird.

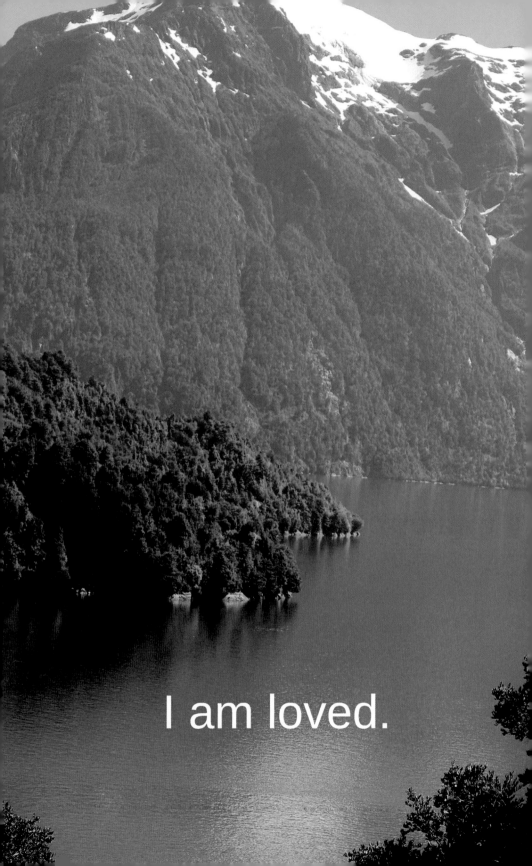

I am loved.

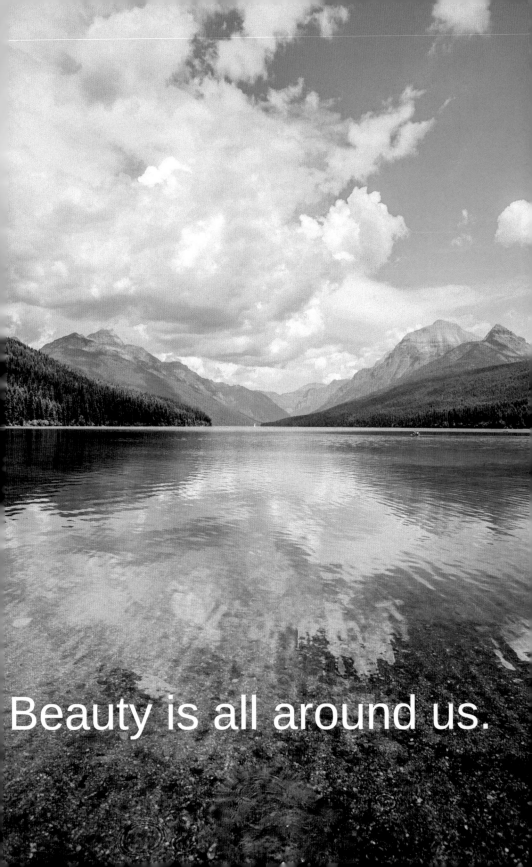
Beauty is all around us.

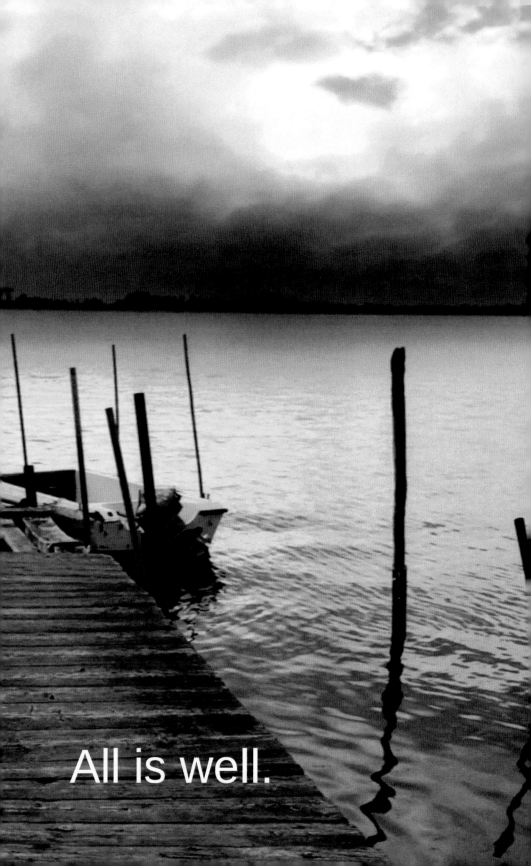

All is well.

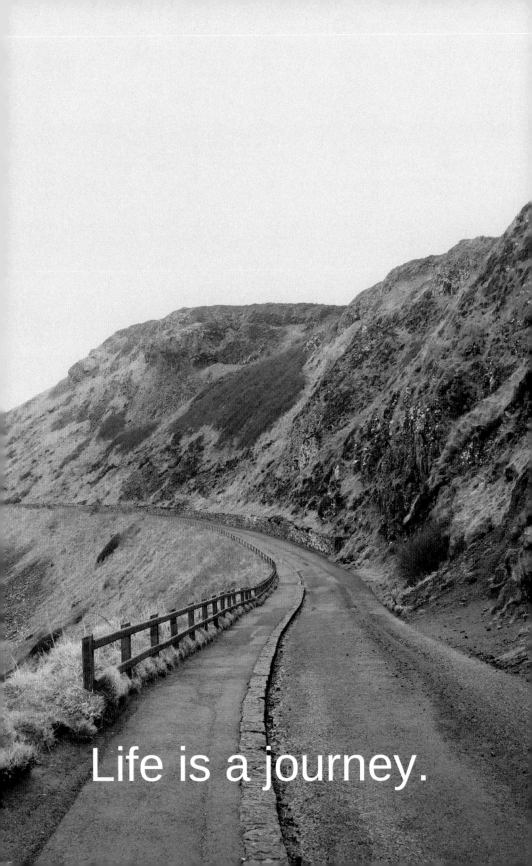

Life is a journey.

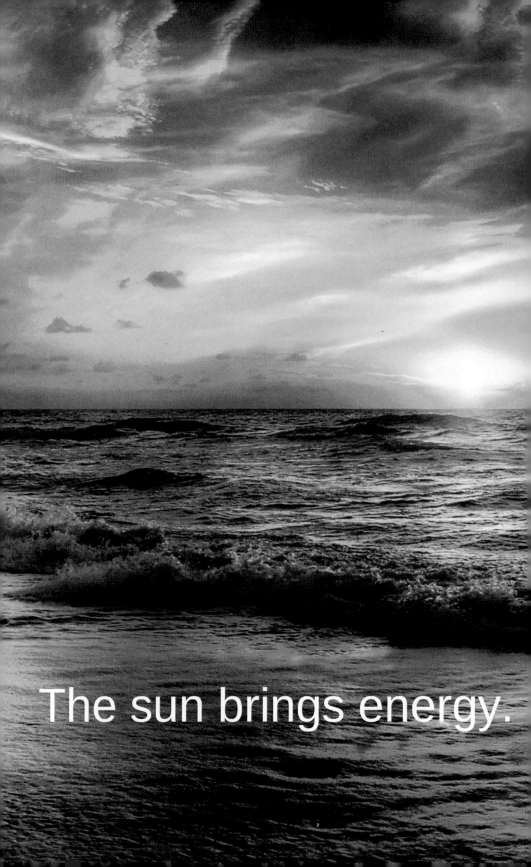

The sun brings energy.

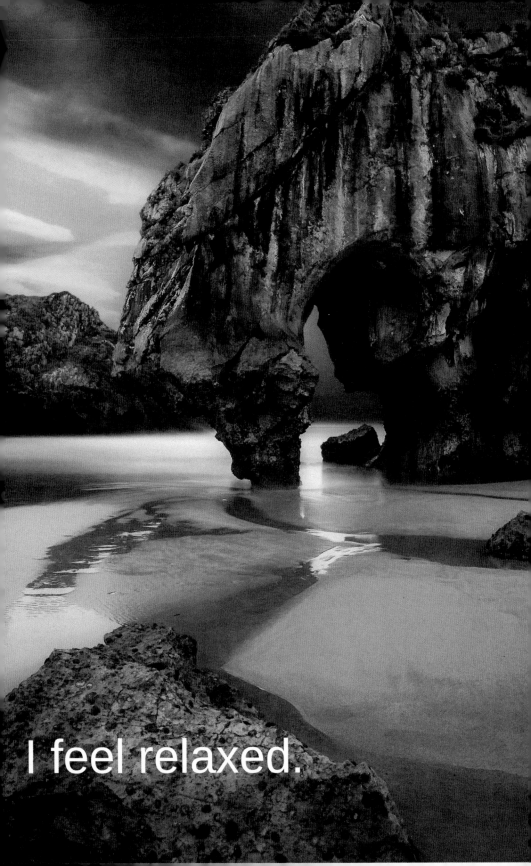

I feel relaxed.

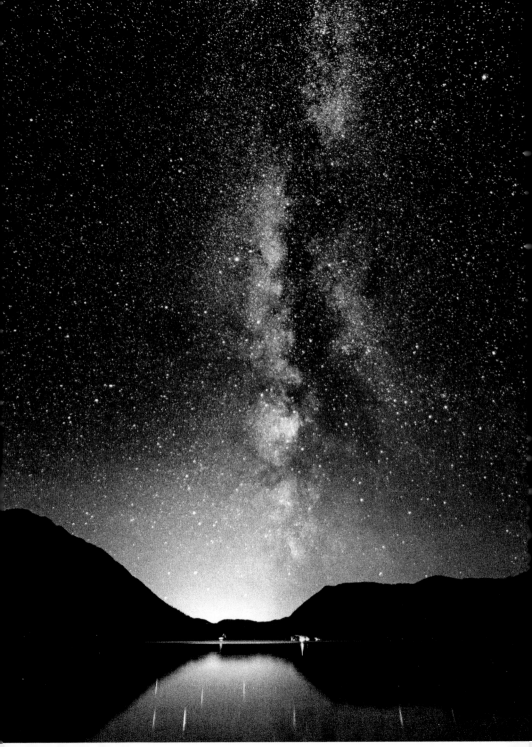

The Earth is beautiful.

Made in the USA
Coppell, TX
09 September 2020